THE FOETAL CIRCULATION

6ᵗʰ and final edition

Alan Gilchrist

AuthorHouse™ UK
1663 Liberty Drive
Bloomington, IN 47403 USA
www.authorhouse.co.uk
Phone: 0800 047 8203 (Domestic TFN)
+44 1908 723714 (International)

Because of the dynamic nature of the Internet, any web addresses or links contained in this book may have changed
since publication and may no longer be valid. The views expressed in this work are solely those of the author and do not
necessarily reflect the views of the publisher, and the publisher hereby disclaims any responsibility for them.

Any people depicted in stock imagery provided by Getty Images are models,
and such images are being used for illustrative purposes only.
Certain stock imagery © Getty Images.

This book is printed on acid-free paper.

ISBN: 978-1-7283-9505-0 (sc)
ISBN: 978-1-7283-9506-7 (e)

Print information available on the last page.

Published by AuthorHouse 04/22/2020

authorHOUSE®

This little book is dedicated to my
parents, James and Ivy Gilchrist, and to
my wife Pauline.

Acknowledgements

The 5th edition of this book was produced in cramped quarters when I was living with my son Andrew and his wife Kim and their three sons. Since October 2018 I have been living by myself in a little flat which has given me more space to live and work in. Andrew has been a great help in the transition and keeps an eye on me from time to time, while I miss Kim's expertise assistance on my computer. Most important was having the space to fit in a deep freezer in which I could store my animal dissections, instead of just bottling them in formalin and keeping them in the garden. The move seems to have helped me to think more clearly and this final edition introduces many new ideas. In the 5th edition I told you about my back injury which prevented me from working on one of the lambs, but though I am less mobile now I have been able to examine more foetal lambs and complete this edition. I now have a little scooter which is a great boon; I can whizz round to the shops at 3.8 mph and get all I need without waiting for buses. I have tried to improve the quality of my diagrams, but some of the letters of the captions are still wobbly.

I am very grateful to Sophia Anderton, Head of Publishing & Digital Learning in the British Institute of Radiology, who has very kindly permitted me to publish details of two articles from the British Journal of Radiology. To Oswestry farmer Graham Jones, I again give many thanks for providing me with stillborn lambs which have played a large part in helping to unravel the hidden mysteries of the foetal circulation. In this regard I must also thank Kevin Battams of Battams Butchery in Oswestry for providing me with parts of the postnatal lamb. I still run into difficulties with my laptop, but I have been helped at home by Ben Hillidge of the Reliant Company in Oswestry. Nigel of Cartridge World Oswestry has again come to my rescue and solved my printer problems. A special mention and thanks for John Quinn, photographer in Oswestry for the high quality of his work in reproducing my diagrams in high resolution. This little book conceived in Africa and nurtured in England, has been safely delivered after a long and difficult labour, in Oswestry. It is a newly born offspring of Oswestry, which is now able to receive visitors. I invite you to come and see it. Alan.

References

The Foetal Circulation. The Personal Account by a Zimbabwe Family Practitioner. By Alan Gilchrist. Printed in Zimbabwe by Graphtec Zimbabwe.2011.

A Visit to Nyasaland/The Foetal Circulation. By Alan Gilchrist. Printed by YOUCAXTON PUBLICATIONS. 2014.

The Foetal Circulation Reflections. By Alan Gilchrist. Printed by YOUCAXTON PUBLICATIONS. 2015.

The Foetal Circulation. By Alan Gilchrist. Published by AUTHORHOUSE. 2017.

The foetal Circulation. 5th Edition. By Alan Gilchrist. Published by AUTHORHOUSE. 2018.

Foetal and Neonatal Physiology. By G. S. DAWES. Published by YEAR BOOK MEDICAL PUBLISHERS, INC. Chicago. 1968.

Contents

The Foetal Circulation.

Part One

The Plan

In the postnatal creature, which I call a postnate, Diagram 1, the two great arteries which leave the heart together curve upwards; the pulmonary trunk from the right ventricle ending abruptly by bifurcating into the two pulmonary arteries for the lungs, while the aorta from the left ventricle supplies the upper body and curves over the pulmonary arteries to pass down behind them as the descending aorta to supply the lower body.

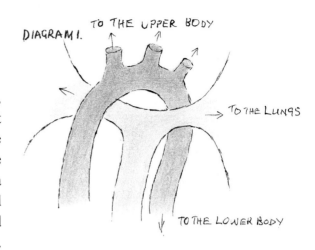

DIAGRAM 1.

TO THE UPPER BODY

TO THE LUNGS

TO THE LOWER BODY

The blood in the postnate is either venous or arterial: venous before it reaches the lungs and arterial afterwards.

In the foetus, Diagram 2, the arrangement is different. The pulmonary trunk extends beyond the pulmonary arteries, supplying them in passing for the unexpanded lungs and ends by joining the aorta. The blood in the descending aorta which supplies the lower body and the placenta is therefore a mixture of venous and arterial.

TO THE UPPER BODY

D 2.

TO THE LOWER BODY AND PLACENTA

D 3.

HEART

INFERIOR VENA CAVA

LIVER

UMBILICAL VEIN

PLACENTA

The re-oxygenated arterial-type blood returning from the placenta in the umbilical vein, reaches the liver and enters the upper part of the inferior vena cava, which carries it to the heart. Diagram 3. According to the orthodox accounts of the foetal circulation, this upper part of the inferior vena cava also carries the venous return from the lower body of the foetus, separated by streaming from the blood from the placenta, and both streams enter the right atrium. The arterial stream is then said to pass through the foramen ovale into the left atrium. Diagram 4.

SUPERIOR VENA CAVA

D 4.

LEFT ATRIUM

RIGHT ATRIUM

LIVER

PLACENTA

INFERIOR VENA CAVA

There is no doubt that some streaming does occur in blood vessels, but not of the respiratory gases in solution. Where there are different levels or pressures of oxygen and carbon-dioxide in solution close together, there is a rapid movement of each gas from higher to lower, resulting in equilibrium and a homogeneous mixture of both, with pressures midway between the two extremes. It is this extremely fast reaction which allows us to carry out the most strenuous of activities in the best of health. There was a very good demonstration of it during the Oxford and Cambridge boat races on 7th April 2019. Some of the crews had sensors on their big toes which recorded their heart rates going up to more than 200 beats per minute. Their respiratory rates were also high, probably approaching the stroke rates of the oars at 40 breaths per minute. The flow of air in the lung airways, and the flow of blood in the capillaries of the lung respiratory zone would pass each other at excessive speeds, and in the briefest moment of time carbon-dioxide would pass from the lungs to the air, and oxygen would pass from the air into the blood. Otherwise all the crews would succumb from oxygen lack and excess carbon-dioxide. And if two separate streams of arterial and venous blood were to enter the foetal inferior vena cava side by side, the same reaction would lead immediately to a mixed homogeneous stream with a low oxygen level and excess carbon-dioxide which would kill the foetus. *Separation of the respiratory gases by streaming cannot occur; it is a myth.* Diagram 5 A. shows the fast reaction. B. shows how two streams side by side quickly become homogeneous.

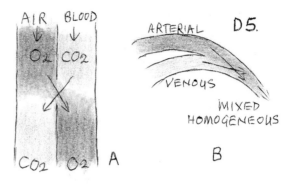

We can therefore rule out any possibility of a venous stream joining the arterial placental stream if the foetus is to remain healthy and there can be only one stream, the placental. We can also be certain that the placental stream would lead to the left atrium; any suggestion of it leading to the right atrium would be absurd. Diagram 6. It is the venous return from the lower body which would lead to the right atrium, but not together with the placental stream. The inferior vena cava must be separated functionally in the region of the liver into two parts: the upper to supply the left atrium and the lower to supply the right, and the lower return must reach the right atrium by an alternative route.

After the placental stream has passed through the left side of the heart it joins the venous flow from the right heart *beyond* the heart, *not proximally,* as I have shown you in diagram 2, and the mixed stream must contain the venous return from both parts of the foetus because all the venous return must be replenished by the placenta. We therefore know that the lower venous return would have already entered the right atrium by an alternative route and joined the upper return. We also know that the mixed blood in the descending aorta would be homogeneous. Diagram 5. B.

Recently I have been able to obtain from the British Institute of Radiology a copy of an article published in the British Journal of Radiology in 1939. Vol. XII, No. 141. It demonstrated with intravascular injections of radio-opaque substances and radiological cinematography, the circulation of the blood in live foetal lambs. It reveals the difficult complicated pioneering work performed by A. E. Barclay, Sir Joseph Barcroft, D. H. Barron and K. J. Franklin, in the Nuffield Institute for Medical Research, Oxford, and shows for the first time, the circulation not only in live foetal lambs with x-rays, but probably in the unborn child without exposure to radiation.

Their work would have been carried out just before the outbreak of the second world war, and we must realise that at that time there was a strict anti-abortion law, with few human foetuses available for research.

Only a year before, an eminent obstetrician had been arrested by the police for terminating the three months' pregnancy in a fourteen- year old girl who had been raped by five British soldiers. The Oxford work would have been a landmark in the investigation of the foetus, and the results would have been accepted as the norm. The quality of the work was of the highest calibre, and the photographs they have allowed us to see are very valuable, but the conclusions reached were mainly wrong.

Many of the pictures show radio-opaque material flowing down the superior vena cava to the right atrium. But there is one which shows the same sort of material flowing up the inferior vena cava. The article says: 'In the foetus, the inferior caval flow is composed of oxygenated blood returning to the heart from the placenta *via* the umbilical vein, and venous blood from the lower segment.' This is an assumption; they could only be certain that the blood flowing up the inferior vena cava contained the oxygenated blood from the placenta. It then says: 'We have not as yet traced the course taken by this venous blood, our experiments having been confined to the demonstration of the flow from the umbilical vein.' It continues: 'The main portion of this stream, after entering the right auricle, passes through the foramen ovale to the left auricle and left ventricle.' (The word 'auricle' is now no longer used and has been substituted by 'atrium'). This is another assumption. It is quite impossible to make out the details of the atria, and in any case the picture they show is different from the others which do show the right atrium, and therefore the mainstream may have entered the left atrium, not the right.

FIG. 2A.
(Sheep fœtus.) Injection passing down the superior vena cava, through the right side of the heart to the pulmonary trunk, and thence to the pulmonary arteries and (*via* the ductus arteriosus) to the descending aorta. Note the conus arteriosus and pulmonary valve.

FIG. 8A.
(Sheep fœtus.) Radiograph showing an injection passing up the inferior vena cava to the right auricle. The greater part of the contrast medium passes through the foramen ovale to the left side of the heart, and thence to the aorta and brachio-cephalic artery. A small quantity, however, is also seen in the right side of the heart, the pulmonary trunk, and the ductus.

I am grateful to the authors for having shown the results of their work; the pictures are quite extraordinary and allow me to draw my own conclusions, which differ from theirs. I have introduced two photographs here. The first shows the opaque material flowing down the superior vena cava to the right atrium, while the second shows the injection flowing up the inferior vena cava. They say this flow in the inferior vena cava goes to the right auricle, but as I have said earlier, it can only go to the left atrium. Further on they say: 'In addition, however, a certain quantity is detached from the main stream in the right auricle and is carried through the right atrio-ventricular (tricuspid) valve to the right ventricle and pulmonary trunk.' There is no mention of streaming here, but is it not inferred? Earlier in the article the authors point out that none of the blood from the superior vena cava which enters the right atrium passes through the foramen ovale, but the blood which enters the right atrium from the inferior vena cava does pass through the foramen ovale. This suggests to me that these two 'right' atria are two different atria, and that the blood from the inferior vena cava may not have entered the right atrium, but the left. The authors are in fact saying that all three streams leading to the heart enter the right atrium, with no stream leading directly to the left. Perhaps this was the origin of the preposterous concept of right heart dominance, for which there was no evidence.

Although this article revealed parts of the foetal circulation which confirmed what was known, it failed to identify the unknown vitally important features which are necessary to understand it all. It seems to me that the authors were more intent on confirming the old wrong orthodox ideas rather than challenging them. At the beginning they say: 'the object of the foramen ovale is to allow re-oxygenated blood from the placenta to pass from the right auricle to the left side of the heart.' *This is the fundamental error of the orthodox accounts,* as I will show later. It is a pity that they did not complete their investigation of the venous flow in the lower segment of the inferior vena cava; it may have solved many of the problems. Their work was of the highest quality, but not sensitive enough to discriminate between some parts of the heart chambers and the vessels and has several misleading assumptions.

In 1968 G. S. Dawes produced a book called 'Foetal and Neonatal Physiology', published by Year Book Medical Publishers, INC. Chicago, which held the copyright. With some difficulty I have been able to get a copy. It appears that Geoffrey Dawes would have devoted much of his professional life to the investigation of the foetus, and the book covers it in depth from many angles. The results of his work were based on his investigations, also carried out in the Nuffield Institute for Medical Research in Oxford, and he used the same technique of cineangiography on live foetal lambs used by the previous Oxford group. I have been unable to trace the present owners of the copyright of this book, if there are any, so I am not allowed to discuss in detail its contents. However, I can say that as regards the plan of the circulation, his work was inferior to the earlier Oxford work because he does not show us his photographs, *only diagrams of his conclusions,* which are quite bizarre and awfully wrong. There is a good example on the outside front cover of the book. He appears to have laboured all along under the fundamental misconceptions of the plan, as his predecessors had done; which is a pity, because his ideas are still quoted as the orthodox in standard medical publications. I am able to condemn with confidence the conclusions of both Oxford researches, because of some of my own investigations carried out in Africa some fifty or so years ago, supported by animal dissections performed more recently in England.

Since my student days I had been concerned how two streams of blood: one arterial and the other venous, could enter the same chamber of the heart and remain separate. Then in 1965 when I was working in the Fort Victoria hospital in Rhodesia, I was given the answer. (In 1980 Rhodesia became the independent country of Zimbabwe, and Fort Victoria was re-named Mazvingo). For three out of the four years spent there I was single-handed. Then, as well as caring for the hospital patients, I became involved with a huge amount of forensic work for the police. Every few days, or even daily, a police Land Rover with an aluminium coffin on its roof would drive up with a body for me to examine. I sometimes spent more time in the mortuary than in the wards. The clinical work on the one hand and the forensic cases on the other combined to make the whole a unique medical experience without equal: four years of forensic medicine side by side with four years of clinical medicine of great diversity. I have not told you these things only to show you some of the interesting happenings of that time, though they are interesting; I was now doing the work of a forensic pathologist, and it was the work in the mortuary which led to my solving the riddle of the two streams in the right atrium.

In April 1965 a baby girl was delivered in the hospital under my care and died because we were unable to make her breathe. Her body had been taken to the hospital mortuary, where not surprisingly I was performing a police post-mortem. I was engrossed in my work, but my thoughts gradually turned to her. If she had not breathed, would she have been like a foetus which does not breathe in utero, and would her circulation still be in the foetal condition? I finished the post-mortem, went over to her and opened her chest. The heart lay horizontally above the raised diaphragm with the unexpanded lungs on each side. It is a very strange thing; none of the accounts I have read mentions the raised diaphragm and the position of the thoracic organs. I assume it is the normal arrangement contributing to the economy of space, so important in the little curled up intrauterine creature. Diagram 7.

I removed the heart and lungs together, put them in preserving fluid, took them home and later examined them.

Straight away I could see how the streams were separated. It was an emotional moment for me; the first time I had examined a foetal heart which gave me the answer I was seeking. Why had it not been revealed before? I cast my eyes upwards. Had I been guided? The mouth of the inferior vena cava, which was oval, did lead to the right atrium, but not into it. Instead it was closely and accurately applied round the foramen ovale in the atrial septum and led into the *left* atrium, not the right, and in life the placental flow would have entered the *left* atrium without having entered the right atrium at all. Diagram 8. The wall of the right atrium was folded inward, making a tube which ran above the inferior vena cava from the superior vena cava to the right ventricle, and in life the venous return in the right atrium would have flowed above the placental stream below. Diagram 9.

The streams are therefore separated because only one of them, the venous stream from the superior vena cava, enters the right atrium. The arterial placental stream in the inferior vena cava leads into the *left* atrium below the other, ensuring that inter-atrial flow does not occur. *Now we see the fundamental error in the orthodox accounts: whether it be from the lungs of the baby or the placenta of the foetus, the oxygen from the respiratory organ goes directly to the left atrium. It is a principle.*

There was a groove between the tubular right atrium and the inferior vena cava which was the sulcus terminalis. When I looked at the upper end of the tube, I could see muscular flaps arranged radially inside it. I opened the tube: the flaps were the musculi pectinati. Diagram 10.

There was a thickened bar of tissue running down the tube opposite the sulcus terminalis, which was the crista terminalis. It ran along the top of the inferior vena cava giving support to that vessel in its contact with the atrial septum. I imagined the cardiac impulse from the pacemaker near the upper end of the crista spreading down the tube, causing the flaps to contract rhythmically in waves and milking the blood down to the right ventricle above the placental stream below. Diagram 11.

I made accurate drawings of the specimen, then showed it to Pauline and explained how the two streams were separated. She said: "It's like a flyover." Now I hadn't thought of that. What an apt description. Diagrams 8-11.

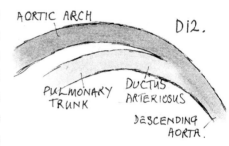

After leaving the flyover the two streams enter their respective ventricles and the arterial is pumped into the aorta, while the venous enters the pulmonary trunk, the end of which is known as the ductus arteriosus. They then meet at the aorto-ductal junction, which I call the junction. Now, I had been concerned about the way the ductus is shown in various articles to enter the aorta. I had imagined it to be a sort of 'T' junction, and after solving the riddle of the two streams I paid special attention to the junction and found that the ductus did not enter the aorta; there was no 'T' junction. That is only a representation of it after birth, when the ductus has closed and shrunk. The ductus was a large vessel, as large as the aorta, and the two vessels lay side by side with a narrow angle between them, converging and joining together to form the beginning of the descending aorta. Diagram 12.

What are we to make of these findings?

1) They confirm what I have said earlier, that the upper part of the inferior vena cava carrying blood from the placenta enters the left atrium.

2) Venous blood from the superior vena cava enters the right atrium.

3) The ductus arteriosus does not enter the aorta.

4) We still do not know the path taken by the venous flow in the lower part of the inferior vena cava. But it cannot join the placental flow, either separated by streaming or as part of a mixed homogeneous stream, and therefore *must take an alternative route.*

In May 1967 I was posted from Fort Victoria to Salisbury, which is now called Harare, and worked mainly in the large Harare Hospital. This turned out to be a very good move with many benefits for the family, and for me a deeper understanding of the foetal circulation. Saturday morning clinical meetings were held in Harare hospital and I gave four presentations: the first on 24th February 1968 was about my observations on the foetal heart. It led to my being invited to examine human foetuses in our medical school.

The first thing I did in the anatomy department, was to examine a foetal right atrium and look for the inferior vena cava attached to the septum round the foramen ovale. But I did not find it; the vena cava led into the right atrium, as it does in the postnate. Without doubt it was a foetus because it had not breathed, and the thoracic organs were closely packed together in the foetal condition. In the other specimens I examined I found the same arrangement. The right atrium in each of these specimens must have unrolled spontaneously either in utero or afterwards, and I presume that at the moment of death, without a cardiac impulse from the pacemaker, the flaccid right atrium may have fallen away from the septum and revealed the postnatal position. Diagram 13. In which case the other investigators could have been forgiven for assuming that the inferior vena cava led into the right atrium

I turned my attention to the foramen ovale and found that it was not a 'little flap valve' as described in some accounts. The name means an oval hole, but when we talk about it, we mean the hole and the parts which cover the hole; the two are synonymous. It consists of two septa: primum and secundum guarding the entrance to the left atrium like the Pillars of Hercules, fused together below and separated above, movement between them allowing blood to pass into the left atrium. The oval hole is the cut-out part of septum secundum facing the right atrium, covered by septum primum facing the left atrium. Diagram 14.

I have three drawings of the valve made in 1968. 'A' shows the valve in the medial wall of the right atrium. 'B' shows the interior of the left atrium, with the atrioventricular opening on the left and the valve on the right. 'C' gives a good view of septum primum in the medial wall of the left atrium, with the upper part of secundum beyond.

It would seem obvious from these drawings that the blood entering the left atrium would have come from the right atrium, but with the atria beating together at the same time there could not have been a flow between them. The authors of the orthodox accounts may have recognised this difficulty, because they say the blood flows through, passes through or is shunted through from high pressure in the right atrium to lower pressure in the left atrium; even though the valve would seem to be designed to prevent backflow from a higher pressure in the left atrium. Now we see the importance of my findings in that little girl's heart, which showed the inferior vena cava covering the valve in the atrial septum and leading the placental flow directly into the left atrium without entering the right atrium at all.

During my work at the medical school I kept my drawings made in 1965 in a nearby cupboard. They disappeared and I do not have a permanent record of my original findings; my diagrams of them here have been made from memory.

I paid a visit to the library of our University Veterinary School. I wanted to see if mammals other than the human had a foramen ovale and musculi pectinati. I thought they must have, but I wanted to confirm it. I read books on the anatomy of the horse, dog and pig. Each one of them had those two features, but there was a third structure common to all of them and to the human. I wondered why those 'lower' creatures should have what we have in our anatomy; was it important? Then I realised its true function in the foetal circulation of us all. *It was the azygos vein.* This vessel connects the two venae cavae and *would serve as the alternative pathway* for the lower venous return to reach the right atrium through the superior vena cava, if the inferior vena cava is blocked to prevent contamination of the arterial stream for the left atrium. Diagram 15.

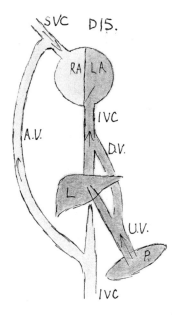

A V= Azygos Vein, D V= Ductus Venosus, I V C= Inferior Vena Cava, L= Liver, L A= Left Atrium, P= Placenta, R A= Right Atrium, S V C= Superior Vena Cava.

No one would deny the importance of the foramen ovale in allowing the placental stream to enter the left atrium. But what about the other feature never mentioned in the orthodox accounts which I read about in the Veterinary School Library: the musculi pectinati? Are they not important? Let us have a look at them. The right atrium is in two parts: a smooth upper part developed from the primitive sinus venosus, and a lower muscular part containing the musculi pectinati originating in the primitive atrium. Blood is collected in the smooth part and pumped into the right ventricle by the muscular part. The musculi seem to be an integral part of the pumping mechanism. In the postnate the total venous return enters the right atrium through two venae cavae at a relatively low rate of about seventy beats per minute. But in the foetus, if I am correct about the alternative pathway, the superior vena cava would carry the total return at twice that speed, and in the rolled up shape of the right atrium the musculi would be closer together and form a more efficient pump to manage this part of the circulation, with perhaps the more subsidiary role of aiding the flow in the postnate. If the superior vena cava does carry all the venous return to the right atrium, it would be one of the reasons for the fast foetal heart rate; there may be others. The musculi pectinati are important; upon their healthy functioning depends the future of the human race, and of all those other creatures which possess them.

At the end of 1969 I resigned from the government medical service, and in April the following year opened my own medical practice in Greendale, leaving the university work and putting off further investigation of the foetus till another day. This came much later than I had expected, and in 2004, when I had become an octogenarian and my practice had become quieter, it began to occupy my mind more and more. In 2011 I produced my own little book. The observations were valuable; some of my opinions questionable. But it was a start, and if I had not begun then I might not have reached the present position, where I have been able to explore and develop my ideas further. In 2013 Pauline died, and I returned to England, where

I have continued to write new versions of my book. What I need to make my work more acceptable and to follow up on the work I had begun in Africa, is to examine more human foetuses, but this has been denied me; I am not allowed to dissect them at home. However, I have been fortunate in being able to make other important observations, as I will shortly reveal.

Since finding the foetal heart in the mortuary I had believed that it is the *foetus* which is delivered, and that the foetus changes into a baby *after* the delivery when the first deep breath is taken. So I was very interested in a programme on television which showed the birth of a foal, and I followed it very carefully. At first, the non-breathing lifeless-looking form of the animal with a narrow unexpanded chest, was delivered on to the ground. Then almost immediately it took a deep breath, opened its chest, stood up on all four legs and shook itself. My belief was confirmed; I had seen a foetus change into a foal. In another programme on television I watched the delivery of a goat kid. It emerged in a flaccid lifeless form and did not breathe. It was still born, and I knew I had watched the delivery of a foetus.

I then realised that stillborn farm animals could be a valuable source of information on the foetal circulation if human foetuses were unavailable, and in February 2018, during the lambing season, Graham Jones, a sheep farmer near Oswestry, kindly gave me four stillborn lambs. The little 'girl' in the mortuary had not been stillborn; she had been delivered alive and had died afterwards. Hers was therefore a neonatal death, but it is the failure to breathe which is common to both the stillborn and the apnoeic neonatal death, and in each case the circulation would not have changed from the foetal to that of a baby. By January 2018 I had completed the manuscript for the 5th edition of my book, but I had to rewrite much of it in February after examining the stillborn foetal lambs.

This year, 2019, I have been able to examine two more foetal lambs, again supplied by Graham Jones. I examined the whole length of an inferior vena cava and could not find a block or an azygos vein. However, in the human foetus and in the horse, dog and pig there is an azygos vein, and I presume there are other alternative routes for the lower return to reach the right atrium in the foetal lamb. In which case the inferior vena cava would be divided into two sections: the lower to carry the lower venous return to the right atrium, and the upper to carry the placental stream to the left atrium. Strictly speaking the upper section should not be called a vena cava because it carries arterial blood to the left atrium and should be given a new name.

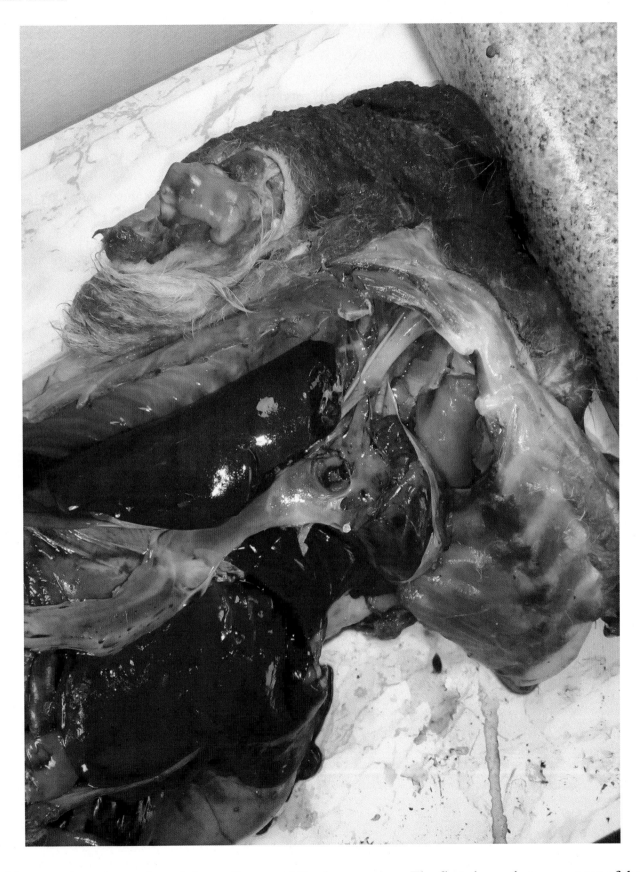

There are four pictures here, taken with my mobile phone camera. The first shows the narrowness of the foetal lamb's chest. In the second the inferior vena cava leads from the liver to the heart. In the third, which I have inverted, I have opened the vena cava and shown how it leads directly to the foramen ovale and left atrium at the far end. The last picture, which I have enlarged, is very revealing: it shows clearly all the details of this section of the circulation. Branching off the inferior vena cava just before it reaches the foramen ovale is a channel leading to the right atrium which has been opened and shows the end of the channel above the opening of the coronary sinus. Between these two features is a crescentic blade which probably helps to convert each into a valve and prevent backflow in atrial systole. Diagram 16 helps to explain.

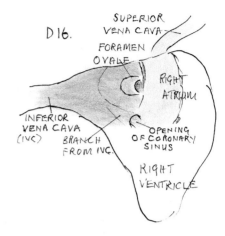

This pre-terminal branch of the inferior vena cava is very important: it provides oxygen and food for the foetal lungs. In the postnate the capillaries of the respiratory zone are the first to receive oxygen from the air in the closely adjacent lung airways, but the non-functional foetal lungs have no access to air. This branch provides them with oxygen and food from the placental stream in the inferior vena cava, which leads blood not only to the right atrium, right ventricle and the pulmonary trunk, but to the pulmonary arteries and the respiratory capillaries in the respiratory zone. It is an unusual arrangement for the lungs, with the pulmonary arteries bringing in oxygen instead of carbon dioxide, and the pulmonary veins returning to the left atrium with carbon dioxide instead of oxygen. There may be an important subsidiary function for the pulmonary circulation: to maintain the flow and prepare the vessels for the moment at birth when all the venous blood will pass through them. Without this branch there would be no lungs, no people, no mammals, and perhaps no birds. This branch and its terminal valve deserve names. Diagram 17.

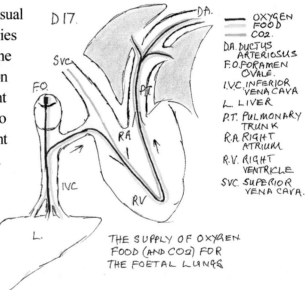

Diagram 18 again shows how the oxygen from the placenta and inferior vena cava reaches the lungs.

Interestingly, the Oxford team had identified this stream of blood for the lungs, in spite of getting some of their anatomical facts wrong. Referring back to the sentence, part of which I have already quoted, they say 'In addition, however, a certain quantity is detached from the mainstream in the right auricle and is carried through the right atrio-ventricular (tricuspid) valve to the right ventricle and pulmonary trunk. Hence, we see a relatively faint shadow in the right side of the heart and pulmonary arteries, *i.e.,* the flow is comparatively small in relation to the mainstream through the left side of the heart and aortic valve.' The 'certain quantity' is not detached *in* the right atrium, it is detached from the mainstream inferior vena cava outside the atrium and then *enters* the right atrium.

In another article from the British Journal of Radiology, Vol XV, No. 177, by A. E. Barclay, K. J. Franklin and M. M. L. Prichard, the authors have introduced their own names for two structures: the *crista dividens* and the *crista interveniens.* The first refers to the 'V' shaped branching of the vessel from the inferior vena cava, while the second appears to refer to the crescentic blade between the end of this vessel and the opening of the coronary sinus.

In 2018 I had traced the umbilical vein to the liver and followed its branches within the liver, without finding a ductus venosus. This year I examined the liver more carefully after it had been hardened in formalin. I spent all day meticulously picking off the parenchyma from the vessels with my dissecting forceps. The umbilical vein entered the left side of the liver. It then arrived at a distribution centre from where branches spread out to every part of the liver. There was a large branch leading across to the right side, with smaller branches being given off along the way. There was another large branch leading to the south west, connecting with the portal vein near the gall bladder. Diagram 19.

I started to uncover the tributaries and trunks of the hepatic veins. There were two large main trunks at the top edge of the liver, with a smaller one between them; I had severed them all from the inferior vena cava when I removed the liver. I followed the smaller one down and traced it to the distribution centre. I exposed the whole channel cleanly then opened it. *It was the ductus venosus inside the liver.* Picture 5.

My examination of the foetal lambs revealed several features. a) It confirmed again that the upper part of the inferior vena cava leads directly to the foramen ovale and the left atrium. b) It

identified the pre-terminal branch from the vena cava for the blood supply of the lungs. c) It demonstrated the distribution of the placental blood supply for the foetal liver. d) It showed how the ductus venosus within the liver carries the placental stream into the inferior vena cava. I have proposed that the upper vena cava should be given a new name, and that its pre-terminal branch and valve should be given names. Once the names have been given, much of the confusion which has surrounded this part of the foetal circulation for so long will have disappeared, but a picture or a diagram such as the ones I have given will always be a helpful accompaniment.

We can now make a plan of the foetal circulation. Diagram 20.

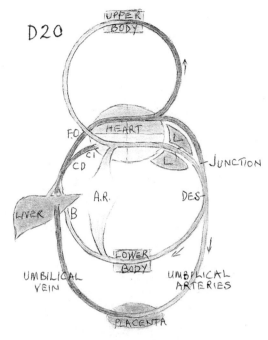

AR= ALTERNATIVE ROUTE B=BLOCK
CD= CRISTA DIVIDENS. CI= CRISTA INTERVENIENS
DES= DESCENDING AORTA. FO= FLYOVER AND
FORAMEN OVALE. L= LUNG.

In diagram 21, I have introduced a different plan of the circulation which separates the heart into its two sides. They are normally joined as one because the right side shares the coronary arterial supply from the left, the coronary venous drainage of the left empties into the right, and both share the impulses from the pacemaker in the right. I have again separated the foetus into upper and lower parts. Although the blood stream in the descending aorta is mixed homogeneous, I have separated the component parts into arterial and venous to make things clearer. The alternative route may be the azygos vein or other vessels.

The first thing we see is the difference between the arterial blood supplies for the two parts of the foetus, with the venous drainage of both leading to the right atrium. Clearly seen is the path taken

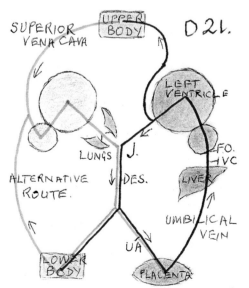

DES= DESCENDING AORTA. FO= FORAMEN
OVALE. IVC= INFERIOR VENACAVA. J=JUNCTION
UA= UMBILICAL ARTERIES.

by the total venous return to the placenta. The amount reaching the placenta must equal the total return from the foetus or the circulation would not be sustainable. The venous supply for the lower body would therefore be an additional supply which has not participated in the metabolism of the foetus, and which could only have come from the metabolism of the lungs. The total disposal of the carbon dioxide (CO_2), has therefore two pathways: the major one from the foetal body to the placenta, and a minor one from the lungs to the lower foetal body. The latter will equate to the amount of oxygen supplied to the lungs from the inferior vena cava at the crista dividens, and the CO_2 leaving the lungs in the pulmonary veins will pass through the left atrium and contaminate the arterial supply for the upper body before reaching the mixed stream in the descending aorta. The venous blood returning from the lower body consists of two portions: one from the metabolism of the lower body and one from the metabolism of the lungs. The arterial blood returning from the placenta also consists of two portions: one from the metabolism of the foetus and the other from the metabolism of the placenta. *Vide infra: The Circulation for the Placenta.*

Part Two

The Sections

The Venturi.

I had often driven through a road junction in Harare where two lanes of traffic converged into one, and the speed of the vehicles in the single lane ahead was twice the speed of the double stream behind. Diagram 22.

This reminded me of the junction in the foetus where two streams joined into one, and I assumed the speed of the blood flowing down the descending aorta after the junction would be twice as fast as the speed in each of the streams meeting at the junction. This is part of the Venturi Principle or Effect, which concerns the increased speed and lowered pressure in a stream of liquid flowing through a narrow section of a tube. (Giovanni Venturi 1797). The junction would therefore segregate the blood supply of the upper body of the foetus coming off the aorta before the junction, from the supply for the lower body and placenta coming off the descending aorta. That for the upper body would be at high pressure, with a full complement of oxygen and food, low in carbon-dioxide and waste, flowing at a certain speed. The mixed stream beyond the junction for the lower body and placenta would be at lower pressure, with less oxygen and food, an increased amount of carbon dioxide and waste, flowing faster than the other.

On 30th March 2019 I removed part of the second lamb which I had kept in formalin, and with my mini Vernier calliper measured the diameters of the vessels before and after the junction. The aorta before the junction measured 22mm, the pulmonary trunk 20.6mm and the descending aorta 26.6mm. The corresponding cross section areas would have been; aorta 363 square mm, pulmonary trunk 318 square mm, and descending aorta 530 square mm. The total area of the aorta and trunk before the junction would have been 681 sq.mm, and the reduction of area in the descending aorta 151 sq.mm. This is a reduction of 22.17%, and the increase of speed would be the same figure; not 100%. Note the similarity of the sizes of the two vessels before the junction, which would indicate a 50/50 mixture of arterial and venous approximately.

The Circulation for the Upper Body.

Diagram 23 The upper body of the human foetus is supplied by three arteries, apart from the coronary arteries for the heart. In the lamb there is only one, which I have called 'cephalic.' The Oxford team called it 'brachiocephalic,' which is more appropriate, because it feeds the forelimbs as well as the head and neck. The arteries in each case come off the aortic arch between the flyover and the junction. It is the most important part of the circulation for the foetus, with a rich supply of

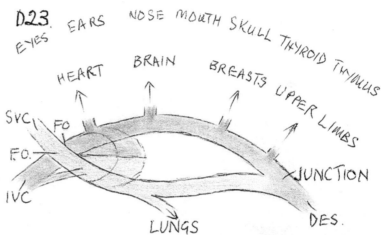

oxygen almost free from carbon-dioxide for many privileged structures on the upper route, which shows the importance of them in the assembly of the new creature. The venous return from the upper body flows in the superior vena cava to the right atrium, as I have shown earlier.

The Circulation for the Placenta.

The junction is a remarkable feature, where two different streams of similar size meet and send mixed blood to the placenta and lower body. The mixed stream for the placenta begins in the internal iliac arteries, and branching off them are the umbilical arteries, which ascend on the abdominal wall to the umbilicus then travel outside the foetus to the placenta. Diagram 24 shows the plan of the vessels but is misleading; the umbilical arteries do not pass downwards. Diagram 25 is more accurate and shows how the blood will circulate. I expect by now you can understand the circulation, and therefore there is no need to clutter up the diagram with letters and directions. The dotted uncoloured circle represents the central left atrium behind the right heart.

The plan of the foetal circulation we have inherited is similar to that of the baby and is just as beautifully simple; but it has been represented falsely as an ugly and complicated one. *It is the similarity of the simple designs of the foetus and the baby which allows the one to change into the other at the very moment of birth.*

The placenta is in two parts: a foetal part which receives the umbilical arteries and a maternal part supplied by the uterine arteries, with the interface between them across which the respiratory gases, food and waste can pass in solution. The arterial portion of the mixed flow to the placenta is probably for the nutrition of the umbilical arteries and those parts of the placenta not supplied by the maternal vessels. As the oxygen of the mixed stream passes through the placenta, it would be used up and replaced by carbon-dioxide, and all the blood reaching the interface would be venous. The maternal side would then receive the carbon-dioxide and waste and give in return to the umbilical vein, oxygen and food: half for the foetus and half for the placenta; probably as quickly as the respiratory exchanges in the boat race crews.

The Circulation for the Lower Body.

We can see why the placenta needs to receive a large flow of venous blood, but why should the venous drainage of the lungs be added to the arterial supply for the lower body? I see it as part of the design which reduces the size of the lower body and the development of the abdominal viscera, the sex organs and the lower limbs, while allowing the heart, the head, the brain and the upper limbs to mature early. The gestation period is also reduced, the head is better shaped and better prepared for the delivery obstetrics, and the hands will be needed early to adjust to the new environment. The abdominal viscera, the sex organs and legs can develop later after birth. Without the venous blood supply, the foetus might have the proportions of an adult, with the mother carrying a monster unable to navigate the birth canal. However, I have not considered the position of the foetal lambs and other quadrupeds which run around with their mothers shortly after birth, with early development of their hind legs, in spite of a 50/50 mixed blood supply. There must be something else to consider.

The venous return from the upper part of the lower body probably travels in the hemiazygos system to the right atrium, while most of the lower return would seem to be diverted to the superior vena cava and join the upper return entering the right atrium.

The Junction.

The junction has been misunderstood and could not have been seen by some of those who have described it. It is often shown with the ductus entering the aorta at a right angle or almost a right angle, Diagram 26 A, and sometimes the ductus is smaller than the aorta, 26 B.

What I saw in 1965 was quite different, as I said earlier. Both vessels were large, of the same size and lay side by side with a small angle between them. They converged together and merged into a single vessel that was the descending aorta. Now we must be quite clear on this point; *neither vessel enters the other.* They lie side by side almost like the twin barrels of a double-barrelled shot gun and *enter the descending aorta together.* Diagram 27.

The two vessels are derivatives of the primitive aortic arches: the aorta from the 4th arch and the pulmonary trunk from the 6th. (The 5th arch is said to disappear completely, but I suspect it may have developed into the two coronary arteries). Diagram 28.

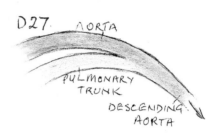

I suppose the concept of a ductus arose because of the mistaken way it was thought to enter the aorta, and it was only natural to think of it as a shunt between the two vessels. In support of these two misconceptions is the anatomy of the junction *after* birth, when the ductus is called the ligamentum arteriosum. The ligamentum does look like a ductus and suggests there would have been a shunt, but in the foetus there is neither. Diagram 29. The concept of a ductus arteriosus leading into the aorta is a complete myth; the primitive arches were never connected like this. However, it needs a name and it is best to retain it, providing that those who do so understand that it lies at the side of the aorta and does not enter it.

The Foramen Ovale.

After birth when the foramen ovale has closed, it becomes converted into a scar known as the fossa ovalis which lies in the septum between the two atria. It has bedevilled us for ages and has suggested that in the foetus, the arterial oxygenated blood from the placenta in the inferior vena cava entered the right atrium and passed through the valve into the left atrium. It could not be pumped through, because the two atria beating together in time on either side of the septum would not be able to propel it through, as I have said earlier. So it was assumed that the pressure in the right atrium was greater than the pressure in the left atrium, and that the blood passed through, entered through, flowed through, was directed through or shunted through; without consideration of the structure of the valve, which appeared to be designed to prevent backflow from a higher pressure in the left atrium to a lower pressure in the right. It was a paradox, an enigma; a riddle unsolved until the death of that little girl in the mortuary in April 1965 which showed that the stream from the placenta in the inferior vena cava led into the *left* atrium, not the right.

The foetal heart has five valves, one more than the postnate; the extra one being the foramen ovale. It is an inlet valve; the only pure inlet valve of the heart. The atrio- ventricular valves are mixed: outlet for the atria and inlet for the ventricles. I believe that inlet valves are opened actively by the muscles attached to them, while outlet valves are opened passively by the weight of the blood pushing the cusps aside. In the condition of atrial fibrillation, the ventricles get little or no help from the atria, and the ventricles do all the work in pumping the blood through the heart. The atrio-ventricular valves, without the atrial component, then become pure inlet valves; opening actively in ventricular diastole, as well as closing actively in ventricular systole. Every person walking around with atrial fibrillation (including myself), is living proof of the ventricles working in ventricular diastole; we cannot live without it. We must therefore abandon the concept of the heart muscles working only in systole and relaxing in diastole. There must be two sets of heart muscle closely apposed: one to contract in ventricular systole while the other relaxes, and the other to contract in ventricular diastole while the first relaxes. (Perhaps we may have to reconsider the interpretation of the electrocardiogram. Could the biphasic RS component be due to the double muscular action I have just described?)

An inlet valve opens in diastole to admit a measured amount of blood and closes in systole to prevent backflow and eject the blood forwards. If we consider the two atria of the foetal heart and the two atria of the postnatal heart, prevention of backflow in atrial systole will be helped in all four by the action of the ventricles in diastole which I have just described, which sucks the blood forwards. The foramen ovale, being an inlet valve, will also strongly prevent backflow from the foetal left atrium when it closes. But the other three atria without inlet valves must prevent backflow in other ways. In the right atrium of the postnate and the foetus it would be important for the sensors of the pacemaker mechanism to have unobstructed access to the venous return from the body. An inlet valve at the entrance to the atrium might be an impediment there, and perhaps, as a compensating feature is the collection of the six valves in the jugular and subclavian veins preventing backflow from the right atrium to the head and neck and the upper limbs. Diagram 30. Also, the milking mechanism which I have described would have a valve-like action, helping to propel the blood forwards.

With the postnatal left atrium, I have considered two factors. The first is the bellows-like action of the lungs, taking in air and blood in inspiration and forcing them out in expiration, expiration taking longer than inspiration. Then there is the backup power of the right ventricle nearby which pumps a continuous flow of venous blood to the lungs throughout the cardiac cycle. But I had overlooked some of my own work which I had carried out in the anatomy department of our medical school. I made several drawings there. One of them, drawing D, taken in 1968 shows the openings of the four pulmonary veins in the area which had been occupied by the foetal left atrium. Three of the openings are oblique and would appear to indicate a valve-like action, preventing backflow into the pulmonary veins in atrial systole. (The fourth cannot be seen properly).

This would apply not only in the foetus when there is a small flow of venous blood from the pulmonary veins into the atrium, but in the postnate too, when all the large inflow would be arterial. I have recently obtained from the butcher a lamb's heart connected to the lungs. There were only two pulmonary veins, one from each lung, and I could not find a valve-like entrance in the wall of the left atrium. However, both entered a recess in the upper part of the atrium close to the auricle, and perhaps in systole that part of the atrium would have contracted and prevented backflow.

In the foetus, the large flow of oxygenated blood enters the left atrium from another direction and gets no help from the non-functioning lungs or the right ventricle. By the time the flow from the two ventricles has passed to the placenta and back to the heart, the pressure in the umbilical vein and the inferior vena cava would be very low; possibly the lowest in the circulation, and the blood supply for the left atrium without an inlet valve would be precarious and haphazard. *The function of the valve is to ensure a constant blood supply for the heart and prevent backflow in systole. It has absolutely nothing to do with shunting blood from one side of the heart to the other.*

On 22nd April 2019, I investigated the foramen ovale from one of the foetal lambs which had been kept in 10% formalin and took many pictures. I first exposed the small unnamed channel which led from the inferior vena cava to the right atrium. I then opened the left atrium and exposed the foramen ovale from the left side. I removed the valve and looked at it carefully from both sides. Round the periphery on both sides was a rim or ring of thickened tissue, and the valve membrane was attached to it. The membrane was flexible and could be folded easily. The top part of the membrane was thickened and anchored at each end. It was a loose membrane which could easily be distended, but not stretched, like a ship's sail which billows out in the wind. The top was crescentic in shape and lay at the far upper end of the inferior vena cava. I tried to work out how the valve would have functioned. In atrial diastole the membrane would have ballooned inwards towards the left atrium, allowing blood to flow through the crescentic gap into the atrium. Then in systole it would have ballooned the other way, pushing the membrane against the atrial wall, closing the gap between the crescent and the ring and preventing backflow into the inferior vena cava.

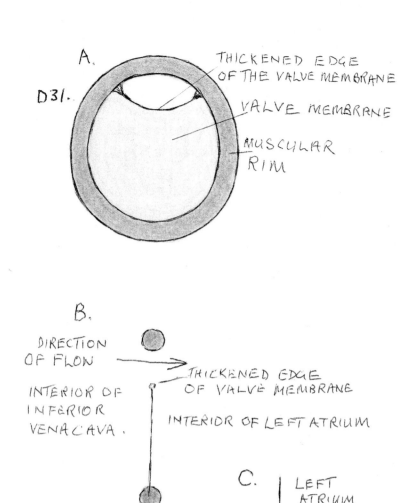

Diagram 31. gives three views of the valve. A. gives a complete view from either side, showing the membrane attached to the muscular rim. In B., I am imagining looking at the edge of the membrane, with the membrane at right angles to my field of vision. C. shows how the edge of the membrane is anchored to the muscular rim; it is a faithful copy of the sketch I made on 22nd April 2019. Note how much thicker is the muscle on the left atrial side.

The next day I blew onto the valve from each side, looking into a mirror held on the opposite side of the valve. When I blew from the vena cava side, I could see the membrane ballooning out beyond the valve, with air escaping easily through the crescentic gap, as blood would have entered the left atrium in atrial diastole. When I blew from the left atrium side the membrane ballooned out into the inferior vena cava side, as it would have done in atrial systole, but the air did not escape through the valve. Instead it escaped outside the valve, on each side across my lips. I then fetched my mobile phone and repeated the blowing onto the valve from both sides, taking pictures with the camera. I enjoyed looking at the pictures, except for my ugly nose of course; it isn't the one I was born with. In May 1961 on a lonely Nyasaland road in the middle of the night, returning to Lilongwe from a court case in Blantyre, I was assaulted by a thug, who clobbered me and knocked me out cold. He damaged my nose and I could not breathe through it properly. A few weeks later I was back in England on home leave. I did not tell my parents about the assault, but while I was sitting in the garden my mother came up to me looking very concerned. She told me how she had woken suddenly in the night a few weeks earlier, sat up and woken my father and said: 'something's happened to Alan.' I had surgery on my nose, and I looked like a rugby player or a boxer who had had a similar operation. I was wrong to blow from the vena cava side; I should have sucked from the left atrium side, to copy what happens in the foetus in atrial diastole. I wanted to do this, again with my camera at the ready, but I could not find the specimen; I must have disposed of it - foolishly.

I investigated the valve further. It had been distorted somewhat by the formalin. The diameter was about 10mm., and the length of the crescentic gap 3mm. I wanted to confirm that the ring/rim of thickened tissue surrounding the membrane was muscle, so I fetched my microscope and examined a small piece; first at times 40, then at times 100, and lastly at times 400 magnifications. The tissue was unstained of course, and a bit dry, but I could easily make out the parallel strips of tissue which ran across my field of vision in a somewhat wavy fashion. I scrutinised them even more carefully and at the highest magnification eventually found some of the strips with barely visible tiny transverse striations. It was muscle: without doubt cardiac! But how would it have functioned during the beating of the left atrium? As I have said previously there must be two sets of cardiac muscle functioning together: one to contract the ring and close the valve in systole, and the other to dilate the ring and suck in blood in diastole. (Somatic muscle is different: the two sets are the protagonists and the antagonists in separate groups of muscle).

Since having examined and drawn the human foramen ovale in the medical school, I had believed that the valve would be an active one, more likely to control the blood flow, rather than a passive little flap blown hither and thither by the blood stream. But what had I found in the foetal lamb but a little flap, not only blown around by the blood, but by my exhaled air too? However, it would be the actions of the muscle of the left atrium which would control the movement of the blood and the valve in diastole and systole. It is all about the directions of the pressure gradients and how they are changed by the actions of the left atrial muscle. Clearly a re-examination of the human valve was a priority, but beyond my reach.

The Left Atrium.

I am re-introducing drawing D which has some interesting features. IA and IV are the abbreviations for the innominate artery and vein, now called brachio-cephalic. A represents the aorta, DA the ductus arteriosus, PA's the pulmonary arteries, PV's the pulmonary veins, and IVC and SVC are the two venae cavae. I have removed the heart from the vessels which pass through the parietal pericardium. Note the difference between the circular muscular aorta and ductus and the flattened venae cavae. The pulmonary arteries arise from the pulmonary trunk proximal to the ductus, so what I have called the ductus is really part of the trunk. It

is as large as the aorta and lies by the side of the aorta without any indication of leading into it.

What interests me particularly is the roughly drawn line round the entrances of the pulmonary veins, which indicates where the attachment of the left atrium would have been. We are never given a good view of the left atrium; it is a central posterior structure of the heart with only the auricle on the left side. But the pulmonary trunk is not part of the heart; it lies above the heart with the pulmonary arteries arising from it. Therefore, in the roots of the lungs, as the pulmonary arteries leave the trunk and the pulmonary veins enter the atrium, the arteries would lie above the veins, close to each of the two main bronchi, as is shown in the anatomy books. Also, as we see from the drawing, the veins would enter the nearest part of the left atrium, the upper part. Notice the position of the inferior vena cava, which shows that the placental stream would have entered the left atrium through the foramen ovale close to the right lower pulmonary vein.

The left atrium is not only a central part of the heart; it is the central part of the circulation in the foetus and the baby. That is why I have illustrated it in an unusual way in my diagrams. In the foetus, the oxygen from the placenta is brought directly to it, and after the oxygen has been distributed to the foetus and the placenta, the blood is returned to the left atrium. We will see later how the constancy of the blood supply for the left atrium is maintained throughout the transition to the baby.

The Postnatal Right Atrium.

I have found it difficult to accept that the respiratory centre in the brain stem could analyse the level of carbon-dioxide in the blood, because its blood supply would have been purified already by passage through the lungs, and it would be protected from the toxic effects of the CO_2. I think there must be a sensory centre proximal to the lungs which can detect the levels of CO_2 in the blood before it has passed through the lungs and relay information to the respiratory centre, which could adjust the respiratory rate to an appropriate level. The system for respiratory control would then consist of three parts: the sensory centre proximal to the lungs, the respiratory centre distal to the lungs, with the lungs in the middle between each. As I see it, the only appropriate place for the detection of the CO_2 levels would be the right atrium, where there is a confluence of all the venous blood arriving from the peripheral tissues. But the pacemaker controlling the cardiac output is also in the right atrium. Is it possible therefore for the right atrium to control not only the cardiac output, but the respiratory rate as well? In which case any activity of the body would be matched by comparable increases in the heart and respiratory rates, under the control of the cardiac and respiratory centres in the brain stem.

The Lungs.

In 1953 I visited the John Hunter Museum in the Royal College of Surgeons in London and saw two beautiful casts of the lungs. The bronchi and pulmonary vessels had been injected with resin and the other tissues had been removed with acid. I noticed a pattern in the relationships between the bronchi and the vessels, but there was no description of it nearby. I have not seen another description of the pattern I had noticed, so I am now describing what I saw in 1953. If you take a key ring and hold it out horizontally, then you can pull a key out on each side. Imagine the keys to be the bronchi painted green, with the pulmonary arteries in blue lying above them and the pulmonary veins in red lying below. Without twisting the keys, you can find the relationship of the bronchi and vessels in any part of the lungs. For example, with the right lung, swing the key up vertically; the pulmonary artery will lie medial to the bronchus and the vein laterally. Swing it down vertically through 180 degrees; the artery will be lateral and the vein medial. Swing it round to the front of the ring; the artery will lie in front of the bronchus with the vein behind. Swing it up through 180 degrees; the artery will lie behind with the vein in front. Swing it round to the back of the ring; the artery will be in front with the vein behind. Swing it down through180 degrees; the artery will be behind with the vein in front. These manoeuvres can be repeated on the left side to give a mirror image of the positions in the right

D32.

ARTERY
BRONCHUS
VEIN

lung. The exercise could be repeated using a small fan, with the unexpanded blades held horizontally with blue paint on the top and red paint below on each blade. Open the fan into a semi-circle and swivel it forwards and backwards with the same result as with the keys. I noticed that the arteries followed this pattern fairly faithfully, but the relationship of the veins to the bronchi was not so constant. In the upper lobes the bronchi and vessels were crowded together, but in the lower lobes there was more space between them. In the upper lobes the arteries would lie central to the bronchi, with the veins lying peripherally. In the lower lobes the arteries would lie on the outside of the bronchi and the veins on the inner side, with a gradual change from above downwards. Diagram 32.

On 25th May 2018, I removed the pleura and lung tissue from the vertebral surface of the lung of a foetal lamb and uncovered the bronchi and vessels. In the upper part the arteries were nearest the surface medially with the bronchi lateral to them. In the middle section the arteries were above the bronchi. In the lowest part the veins were most medial with the bronchi lateral to them. My limited examination of a foetal lung agreed with the arrangement I had seen in the museum. Diagram 33

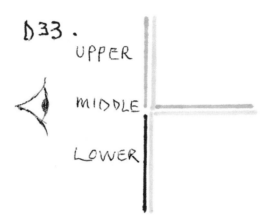

The post-natal lung has a double circulation: a major pulmonary to feed the body with oxygen which drains into the left atrium, and a minor bronchial which feeds the lung with oxygen and drains into the right atrium. The foetal lung is different; the bronchial is dominant because the pulmonary has not opened, except for the diversion of arterial blood from the inferior vena cava for the capillaries of the respiratory zone.

The Liver.

Arterial blood contains food and oxygen. Both are essential for metabolism; one is no good without the other. In the foetus the liver discharges both into the upper part of the inferior vena cava. But in the postnate the liver only discharges food, not oxygen; the oxygen is added in the lungs. Between the liver and the lungs therefore, the blood contains only food and carbon-dioxide, and when the blood reaches the respiratory zone of the lungs an equivalent amount of oxygen is exchanged for the carbon-dioxide.

The Block.

In 1965 I had shown that the upper part of the inferior vena cava led into the left atrium. In 1968 the idea of a block was suggested to me in the Veterinary School library when I read that other mammals had an azygos vein. On page 2, I have shown that the inferior vena cava cannot carry two different streams of blood into the left atrium if the foetus is to remain healthy. Therefore, there can only be the arterial placental stream feeding the left atrium, and the lower venous return must use another route to reach the right atrium. However, the postnatal lower return does use the inferior vena cava to reach the right atrium. There must be an arrangement, a mechanism which guides the lower venous return away from the upper part of the inferior vena cava in the foetus, and at birth there is a change which allows the lower return to use the upper part and flow into the right atrium. I have suggested in all previous versions of my book that there must be a block in the inferior vena cava in the region of the liver, or even in the hepatic cava itself. I have also suggested that the block may be due to the liver being squashed in its cramped quarters high up within the narrow foetal chest, and at birth with the expansion of the chest and the descent of the diaphragm the congested liver would expand and allow unopposed flow in the vena cava. (I have introduced a part of the birth changes prematurely in order to explain these things). In support of these ideas is my limited experience of examining stillborn foetal

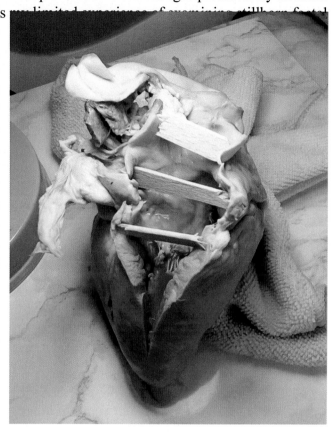

lambs and lambs from my butcher. In 2018, one of the foetal lambs did not have an inferior vena cava below the liver. In the specimen from the butcher which I examined to see the entries of the pulmonary veins into the left atrium, the inferior vena cava was absent completely. In both specimens the lower return must have reached the right atrium by a different route. In the heart without an inferior vena cava the superior vena cava was unusually large. This does not occur in a normal heart because after birth with a slower heart rate the heart gains a second vena cava. But without a second vena cava and with a slower heart rate the heart must have a larger superior vena cava to permit all the venous return to enter the heart.

In this picture I have opened the large superior vena cava in the heart without an inferior vena cava. The right atrium and ventricle have also been opened below it. The fossa ovalis is not well demarcated but can be seen in the atrium between the 2nd and 3rd sticks.

Part Three

The Foetal Heart Sounds

With the long- held view that blood flows through the foramen ovale from the right to left atrium, the valve would be held open, not making a sound until it is closed at birth. But there is a sound as the valve closes with each beat of the heart, as any lady in the later months of pregnancy may confirm with a Doppler foetal heart monitor. The two sounds made by the postnatal heart measure the duration of ventricular systole, with the softer 'lub' heard as the ventricles contract and close the atrioventricular valves, and the harsher 'dup' occurring when the ventricles begin to open and the outlet valves close. The left ventricular sounds are louder than the right sounds, and we need only consider them. The atrioventricular valve is the mitral and the outlet is the aortic. In the foetus there is an extra sound made by the closing of the foramen ovale. It is much softer than the other two and more difficult to hear because atrial muscle is much weaker than ventricular muscle, and when the left atrium contracts in systole the closing valve causes little vibration in the valve and the surrounding blood. But it can be heard nevertheless and occurs just before the other two as the atrium contracts immediately before the onset of ventricular systole. So there will be a triple rhythm; soft lub, louder lub, and harsher dup. Anybody with a Doppler machine should be able to find this rhythm, and it is best not to search for the individual sounds close together at a speed of 140 beats per minute; just find the triple gallop rhythm. Move the machine about and you will find the difference between the double rhythm heard in some places and the gallop rhythm heard elsewhere: diddy-dum, diddy-dum, diddy-dum, with a very short diddy. Diagram 34.

In the fourth version of my book I told you how I had listened to the hearts of the twin foetuses in Emma Pearce and heard the triple rhythm. The sounds were not easily heard because of the small size of the twins. In the 5th edition I described how I had easily heard the heart sounds in Nicola Pilgrim: with triple rhythm on the left side of the abdomen and double rhythm on the right side. It was a single pregnancy, and as it turned out she delivered a fine strong baby boy.

I have often wondered why the sounds should vary between double and triple rhythms. I have some ideas. The left atrium is not left sided, as I have shown in drawing D. It is central and posterior, and the foramen ovale is more on the right side near the right lower pulmonary vein. Is it not more likely therefore, for the sounds to be heard from the back of the foetus, especially as the flexed position of the foetus would keep the front of the chest away from the probing heart monitor?

It was so important to find the triple rhythm; it reveals so much. It shows that the foetal heart has an extra valve, and that it is specifically the left atrium which is beating throughout pregnancy. (The right atrium is beating too of course, but it does not have an inlet valve to contribute to the heart sounds). There must be a flow through the left atrium, *but not from the right atrium:* the flow is from the inferior vena cava as I showed you earlier. You will see later, *in the baby,* when the valve is closed, preventing a flow, that it lies between the atria. The true value of the triple rhythm is therefore to confirm that there is a flow into the left atrium which cannot come from the right atrium; the valve cannot be placed between the atria, and the flow must come from the inferior vena cava. It condemns the orthodox accounts which describe the condition in the baby, with the closed valve between the atria, preventing a flow and not making a third sound.

I sometimes wonder if the triple rhythm can be picked up with a trumpet-like foetal stethoscope. I assume it can, especially by the younger ears of medical students, or by the experienced midwives and obstetricians, if they ever use these useful old-fashioned things. I would be glad to hear from anyone if they have been able to hear the triple rhythm.

Part Four

The Birth Changes

They are in two parts, and both take place outside the mother: the first when the placental circulation is dismantled, and the second when breathing begins.

A bright new light which illuminated the long- hidden secrets of the foetal circulation in April 1965, had been switched on by the death of the little girl who had failed to breathe after her delivery. Why she did not breathe we shall never know, but we will know that the transition from foetus to baby is due to the onset of breathing. The light is never switched on again, and we are kept in the dark during the transition. We can see the external changes: the waking, the breathing and the crying, but the internal changes are shielded from us and have never been seen. But if we have been able to recognise correctly how the foetus differs from the postnate, we will be more able to work out/guess the hidden changes which must occur at birth. As they depend on breathing, they cannot occur in the mother; they take place outside the mother after the delivery. Therefore, the creature which is delivered is a foetus, and the birth of the baby takes place after the delivery on the delivery couch or in the midwife's arms as she is trying to clear the airway, when the first deep breath is taken. The little 'girl' who had died in 1965 would also have been a foetus, and it was her foetal features which had shone so brightly on that April day.

It is important to search for any clues which may help us to understand the internal changes which occur during the transition. But first we must consider the situation of the human foetus to be the same as that of the wild animal foetus, without the presence of any professional medical attendants to affect the outcome of the delivery (apart from the mother). Let us go to the beginning and start with the delivery. As it is completed and the foetus leaves the mother, the emptied contracted uterus will squash the placenta and stop the circulation within it and within all the vessels of the cord, and the foetus will be denied a blood supply. This is a clue; the first evidence of a possible change in the internal circulation of the foetus. There will be a double effect, with the stopping of the flow in the umbilical vein to the foetus, and the stopping of the flow in the umbilical arteries to the placenta. There may be a flow of oxygenated blood into the umbilical vein as the uterus mangles the placenta and wrings out the blood, and this could be of benefit for the foetus at this time if such a flow is able to reach the left atrium, but the loss of the placental circulation heralds the closure of the umbilical vein, with the loss of arterial blood for the liver and left atrium. The effect on the placenta will be more dramatic; there may be pulsation in the umbilical arteries but there can be no flow into the placenta, and the large cardiac output of mixed blood for the placenta will be captured by the foetus and transferred to the lower body. The foetus will therefore gain from the effects on both the umbilical vein and the umbilical arteries and will be well cared for naturally at this time before the delivery of the placenta.

Then the breathing begins. But when does it begin, and why does it begin? It is usually accompanied by the arrival of consciousness; we must not forget that. I believe there must be an inhibitory factor which prevents the foetus from waking and breathing in utero, and that after the delivery it is cancelled, and simultaneously another factor, stimulation, causes the foetus to wake and cry and breathe. The shock of entry into the outside world, with the rapid cooling of the naked wet body of the human foetus like having a cold shower, would seem to be the most obvious external factor. But what about the blocked flow to the placenta? This would be a massive disruption of the circulation, increasing the peripheral resistance at the junction and raising the pressure in the aortic arch and the pulmonary trunk. The large flow of mixed blood for the placenta would be diverted to the lower body in a tsunami-like wave and return as venous blood to the right atrium, spear-headed by the extra venous supply for the lower body. Is it possible therefore, for there to be specific internal factors/triggers which would stimulate the nervous systems of the foetus, and which would inform the foetus when the delivery has been safely completed and when it is safe to wake up and breathe, if the shock of entry into the outside world was insufficient to do so? A sort of fail/safe mechanism.

My account of the birth changes is all guess work, of course, but I have had the benefit of seeing each part of the foetal circulation, which has helped me to work them out. It has not been easy to describe all the many changes because they all happen quickly together at the same time, while I have had to write an orderly description of them one after the other in sequence. They all depend on the expansion of the chest and the descent of the diaphragm when the first deep breath is taken, and all involve the left atrium. Fundamentally they show that the oxygen for the left atrium which had been delivered from the placenta, comes from the lungs as breathing begins at birth. It may not be a single breath, but a series of deep breaths, and especially important is the strong attachment of the inferior vena cava to the central tendon of the diaphragm which ensures that the circulatory and respiratory changes are perfectly synchronised.

The chest has the shape of a cone with the diaphragm rising steeply from its sides to a highly placed central dome, and with the organs packed closely together contributing to the economy of space in the foetus. When the first deep breath is taken the diaphragm and the organs move down to a wider section of the cone, which becomes even wider with the expansion of the chest wall, and there is a sudden increase in the size of the thoracic cage matched by a sudden decrease in intra-thoracic pressure. Two fluid components allow the chest and lungs to expand: air entering the respiratory passages from the trachea, and venous blood diverted from the pulmonary trunk to the pulmonary arteries of the lungs. Both are indispensable and quickly meet each other in the respiratory zone of the lung periphery. The air brings oxygen to the lungs, and the blood will carry the oxygen to every part of the body for all its functions. This diversion of blood to the lungs, the second of the two great diversions during the birth changes, is a major event with a beneficial massive disruption of the circulation. It is the hallmark of the changes, giving the foetus a new life of independence from the mother as it becomes a baby. But all the other changes have happened too. The tissues which separate the inferior vena cava from the right atrium are broken down and the vena cava leads into an enlarged right atrium containing the foramen ovale. The valve now lies between the atria, beating together on each side of it, and without a flow between them the valve becomes functionless and closed, cutting off a supply for the left atrium. The descent of the liver to a wider section of the chest unblocks the inferior vena cava, the right atrium gains a second vena cava and the right atrium receives the venous return from both venae cavae directly which is added to the great diversion, and all the venous blood in the circulation quickly enters the lungs. The diversion suddenly removes the venous blood supply from three parts of the circulation: the ductus arteriosus, the lower body and the placenta. The ductus, lying beyond the origin of the pulmonary arteries, collapses and closes without a venous blood supply, and abolishes the segregated blood supply. The venous portion of the mixed stream for the lower body is replaced immediately by arterial blood, which flows down the descending aorta behind the departing mixed stream. If the first deep breath is taken before the transfer of blood from the placenta to the lower body, most of the blood diverted will be diverted from the placenta, with less from the lower body. But if there is delay in the onset of breathing most of the blood will be diverted from the lower body and less from the placenta. Either way, all the venous blood in the circulation will be diverted to the lungs where it will be oxygenated and flow to the left atrium, left ventricle and aorta, and distributed in full volume to both parts of the body at equalised pressure and speed. It all happens in the twinkling of an eye, invisibly in front of those who are privileged to witness the birth of a waking baby, when the first deep breath is taken.

It is great theatre: the left atrium occupies centre stage, with dissolution and assembly side by side in each wing as the first deep breath is taken. On the right, both venae cavae enter the right atrium directly and the blood is directed into the right ventricle and pulmonary trunk, while the foramen ovale is closed and the left atrium is denied a blood supply. On the left, the blood in the pulmonary trunk is diverted from the lower body and placenta to the lungs and left atrium, with an uninterrupted supply of oxygen for the changing creature, while the ductus arteriosus closes and arterial blood is distributed to both parts of the body equally.

When the first deep *expiration* is taken the organs do not return to their foetal position but take up a new fixed lower position from where all future respiratory excursions will be made. There are other changes too: the heart becomes more vertical and the heart rate is decreased, with loss of the atrial sound and the gallop rhythm. The panicky crying stops as the baby is comforted on the breast, and quiet breathing begins. Very soon there will be a wet or soiled nappy as the three functions of the placenta are taken over by the lungs, the kidneys and the alimentary tract.

Diagram 35 shows how the diversion of the venous blood from the pulmonary trunk to the lungs closes the ductus arteriosus, abolishes segregation and arterial blood is distributed to both parts of the circulation equally. In 'B' we catch the very moment when all the birth changes begin, and the total venous return is directed to the lungs instead of the placenta and lower body.

I was not able to include the bronchi bringing air into the lungs or the pulmonary veins returning with oxygen to the left atrium. But diagram 36 shows how the left atrium is supplied with oxygen in the foetus and the baby. In B, the red shaded areas converging onto the left atrium represent the pulmonary veins bringing in oxygen.

Throughout the life of the foetus and during the transition to the baby, the left atrium and upper body are well supplied with oxygenated blood. The lower body has some changes because of the dismantling of the junction. As I see it, we should consider the Venturi again. In the foetus both ventricles pump strongly against the narrow junction and the pressures in the aorta and pulmonary trunk would be high, while the mixed stream in the descending aorta would be flowing quickly at low pressure. When the venous blood in the trunk is diverted to the lungs the pressure in the aorta would drop and a single stream of arterial blood would flow through the aorta without a narrow obstruction. It would immediately replace the diverted venous flow and flow down the descending aorta at a reduced speed in full volume, at the back of and in continuity with the departing mixed stream. The vessels in the human Venturi are responsive, probably specially designed to adjust to this situation and maintain an adequate circulation in each part.

I want to emphasise three things.

First, that each foetal atrium has only one vena cava: the inferior for the left and the superior for the right. At birth when the diaphragm descends the inferior vena cava switches over to the right atrium, which then receives a second vena cava, while the placental supply for the left atrium is replaced by fresh blood coming from the lungs.

Secondly, the respiratory and circulatory changes at birth are perfectly synchronised because each depends on the descent of the diaphragm. Crucial to the synchronisation is the strong attachment of the inferior vena cava to the central tendon of the diaphragm; it is the place where respiratory and circulatory anatomy and physiology meet, and ensures that the circulatory changes occur at the same time as the onset of breathing. The one cannot occur without the other, and without the descent of the diaphragm neither occurs. That is why the little 'girl' in the mortuary gave up her secrets to me, because the diaphragm had not descended (what an important observation that was), and both her heart and lungs were still in the foetal position.

Thirdly, and most importantly, it is the foetus which is delivered; the baby is born after the delivery when the first deep breath is taken.

Conclusion.

I want to end my story by showing you a picture of part of the anatomy of a lamb. Not a foetal lamb, but a lamb that had been gambolling in the hills round Oswestry for several months before reaching the butcher's shop. It shows the inferior vena cava, propped open with a stick, leading into an enlarged right atrium containing the remains of the foramen ovale, known as the fossa ovalis. This view of the fossa ovalis has bedevilled us for ages, but only because we have allowed it to do so. It has suggested that in the foetus the placental stream in the inferior vena cava led into the right atrium before passing through the foramen ovale into the left atrium. We must not assume the anatomy of the foetus to be the same as that of the postnatal creature without examining the foetus as well.

In the earlier enlarged picture, reduced and reproduced here, I have shown how the upper part of the foetal inferior vena cava is separated from the right atrium and leads the placental stream directly into the left atrium through the foramen ovale, without entering the right atrium at all. *The right atrium has nothing to do with the placental stream; it is the receptacle of the venous return.*

Where there are two pumping chambers in line, for a flow to occur they must beat in sequence; first the one then the other. This is what happens on each side of the heart. If the chambers beat at the same time, there will be no flow between them. This is what happens in the foetus at birth, when the inferior vena cava leads into the right atrium and closes the foramen ovale. When the placental stream leads into the left atrium, flow will occur in atrial diastole because the low positive pressure in the inferior vena cava will be greater than the negative pressure in the atrium. In atrial systole the valve will close, and the blood will be ejected at high pressure into the left ventricle. The concept of blood flowing from the right atrium to the left atrium through the foramen ovale is an impossible, irrational one and quite wrong. Yet it appears throughout all the orthodox accounts.

Alan Gilchrist

There are three valuable pictures here, taken with my mobile phone camera, of foetal lambs' hearts which had been preserved in varying dilutions of formalin.

The first, taken on 7th June 2018 and shown below, is an enlarged reproduction of picture 8 from the 5th edition of this book. The longer stick is in the superior vena cava leading into the right atrium, while the short stick props open the inferior vena cava, which I have cut, and which leads to the foramen ovale at the far end. Branching off the inferior vena cava is the un-named vessel which leads into the right atrium above the opening of the coronary sinus.

The second, quite remarkable picture, taken on 22nd April 2019, shows the inferior vena cava, which I have cut open, branching at the crista dividens into a larger part feeding the foramen ovale on the left, and a smaller part which is the un-named vessel leading into the right atrium on the right.

The third picture, also taken on 22nd April 2019, does not show the branching at the crista dividens so clearly, but gives an excellent view of the crescentic blade, which is the crista interveniens, separating the end of the un-named vessel from the opening of the coronary sinus into the right atrium.

The scar of the foramen ovale, known as the fossa ovalis, includes the scar of the un-named vessel on its right side. On page 31 the bi-part nature of the fossa is shown in the picture taken on 7th July 2018, which is a reproduction of picture 16 from the 5th edition, and which is best seen with a magnifying glass. The un-named vessel is in effect an arterio-venous fistula supplying oxygen and food from the inferior vena cava to the foetal respiratory capillaries.

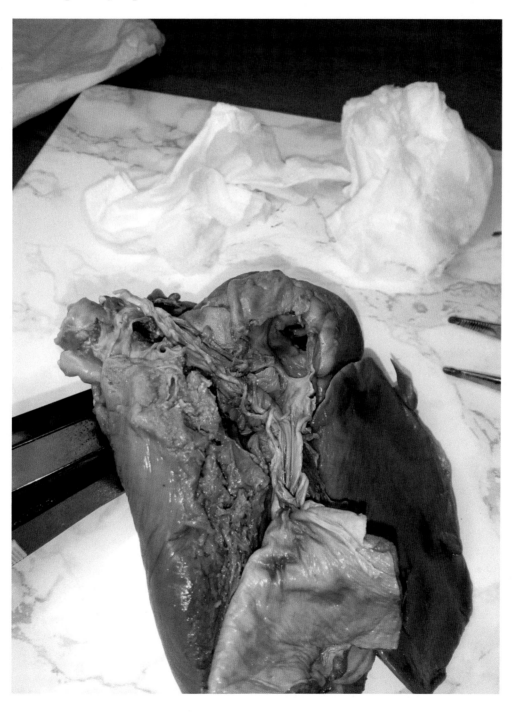

Printed in the United States
By Bookmasters